The information provided in this book is for informational purposes. It should not be used for diagnosing or treating a health problem or a disease without consulting a health professional.

It is not a substitute for professional care. You must consult a health care provider if you suspect that you may have a health problem. The statements that describe the remedies have not been evaluated by the Food and Drug Administration.

Limitation of Liability
This book shall not be liable for any special or consequential damages that result from the use of, or the inability to use, the materials in this book or the performance of the products.

This book is just the tip of the iceberg in herbal remedies. These have been used in our family for years. The best thing to do is find out what your family's needs are and research those issues.

If there is an emergency and no hospital is available, no medical help, are you prepared to help your family in a crisis?
These remedies are a way to buffer between your family and a disaster. For the most part they are gentle, and may work better than modern medicines to some degree, depending on the person.

People tend to forget that modern medicine was derived from the plants, minerals, and nature before it became "modern". Always check with your physician, but the best decision you can make is research, research, research. Start small and as you gain a knowledge, expand. You will be surprised at what you will find.

Chapter One
BEGINNING HERBAL

Do's and Don'ts of Natural remedies:

Do:

- Essential oils store better in dark colored bottles and refrigerated.
- Store all medicines in a cool, dry place.
  Do your research. If something appeals to you, look it up.

- Do not eat or drink 20-30 minutes each side of taking the remedy if oral.
- Keep away from pets and children
- Keep an eye on expiration dates. Make sure remedies are marked clearly with the date made, and date expired.
- Many of the wound treatments work for both human and animal, but make sure you check with a vet before using on your pet or livestock.

Don't

- Don't drink coffee or smoke while taking treatments.
- Unless required in a recipe, don't use the essential oils of camphor, eucalyptus, menthol, peppermint, or rosemary, while taking treatments

General list of Natural Remedies

Activated Charcoal
Reduce inflammation, draw out infections, treat abscesses, infections, boils, burns, gangrene, provides pain relief, relieve itching from bug bites, and is amazing for spider bites. Treats swelling and inflammation from strains, sprains, and tendon injuries.

Cayenne Pepper
Safety issues: Cayenne as a spice is considered safe during pregnancy, but pregnant women should avoid taking Cayenne as a supplement. Cayenne passes into breast milk, so nursing mothers should avoid Cayenne. When taking Cayenne, start with peppers with lower heat gradually working to hotter types. Shock may occur if starting out with extremely hot peppers.
Cayenne pepper, has been used with great success to stop heart attacks in it's tracks before medical help could arrive in areas without doctors. It is also used in treating flatulence, high blood pressure, Diptheria, hemorrhoids, Scarlet Fever, sore throat, sinusitis, nausea, fever, gout and much more.

Chamomile
Safety issues: None
Used for eye infections, toothaches, insomnia, soothes, cuts, burns, dry skin, diaper rash, PMS, all skin conditions including eczema, inflamed skin and infections, sleeplessness and colic in children, and diarrhea.

Comfrey
Safety Issues: Although some uses are taken internally, this author suggests using Comfrey topically, related to possible toxins that may be found in this plant.

Used for wounds, sprains, skins ulcers, joint inflammation bruises, fractures, gout, and Rheumatoid arthritis.

Cloves
Safety Issues: Clove oil must be diluted as it has very strong properties. Should not be used with people who have extremely sensitive skin. Clove oil has been known as blood thinner, so don't use while taking medications that thin the blood. Pregnant women should not use clove oil, and Diabetics should also be very cautious. Clove oil has been known to lower blood sugar.

Clove oil is used for treating a variety of health disorders including toothaches, indigestion, cough, asthma, headache, Cholera, Diabetes, and stress and blood impurities.

Echinacea
Safety Issues: Do not use for more than 10 days in a row. Take a break before using again. Some people may be allergic. Avoid during pregnancy. Studies show it MAY be safe for pregnant women but not enough have been done to be sure.

Echinacea has been used for common colds, flu, immune system deficiencies, Vaginal fungal infections, and upper respiratory infections. Urinary tract infections, bloodstream infections, genital herpes, Strep infections, tonsillitis, and much more.

Elderberries
Safety Issues: Only the juice from the elderberries should be used, as the seeds contain small amounts of poisonous substances. Once cooked the juice is safe.

Used for colds, flu, H1N1, Plague, Upper respiratory, possibly relieves side effects of some cancer treatments,

Eucalyptus
Safety issues: Must not be swallowed-cases of severe internal poisoning have occurred. Safe on the skin or as an inhalation.

Clears colds, blocked noses, sinusitis, chest infections, soothes burns, cuts, wounds and insect bites, eases muscular pains, improves circulation, improves concentration.

Garlic
Safety Issues: Garlic may alter the function on prescription medications. If you are being treated with Blood thinning medications, aspirin, Warfarin, do not use garlic without first speaking to your health care provider. Also people using protease inhibitors, such as HIV treatments should consult a doctor before using garlic.

Used to fight some forms of cancer, antibiotic, anti-fungal, anti-inflammatory, prevents many forms of cancers; colon, stomach, rectal, prostate, and lung. Controls high blood pressure, high cholesterol, heart disease, and hardening of the arteries. Some other treatments may include, treatments of fevers headaches, diabetes, snakebite, stress, liver function, bronchitis, and sinus congestion. Ringworm and jock itch.

Ginger
Safety Issues: Take in low doses. No more than 2 cups of ginger tea a day for 3 days, then take a break. Interacts with blood thinners, diabetes, and high blood pressure medication. Pregnant women check with physician.

Eases indigestion, aches and pains in muscles, improves poor circulation, superb for colds and flu. Also good for Osteoarthritis pain, and Rheumatoid arthritis.

Honey (Raw)
Safety Issues: May not be given to children under 1 year of age. The infant immune system is not mature enough and most physicians agree that it will possibly cause infant botulism, which is a potentially fatal illness. It is considered safe for Pregnant moms and Nursing moms.

Uses: Antibiotic, Antifungal, Immune system booster, anti-cancer, wounds, bedsores, burns, colds, flu, and eye infections.

Lemons
Safety issues: Slightly phototoxic avoid any exposure to strong sunlight or a sunbed for at least 12 hours after application.

Helps build immunity against colds, influenza and other viral infections, detoxifies the system and assists lymphatic drainage, freshens the mind and helps to improve concentration.

Olive Oil or Coconut Oil
Used for dilution of essential oils, or to make treatments.

Onion
Safety Issues: Interacts with Aspirin and Lithium, avoid using together. Onion also decreases blood sugar in diabetics.
Also slows blood clotting so if you are on blood clotting agents, speak with a physican.

Outstanding for colds, flu, Kidney infections, digestion problems, upset stomach, high blood pressure, arteriosclerosis, asthma, dehydration, parasitic worms, Whooping cough, diabetes, sore mouth ulcers, and boils.

Peppermint
Safety issues: If your skin is sensitive, use half the stated drops of peppermint in any recipe due to the menthol content in the oil which can act as an irritant. Tea use regular strength.

Uses: Eases stomach cramps, indigestion, constipation and nausea; helps muscular aches, stiffness, backache; eases headaches and migraine, clears the head and improves concentration. Also helps with weight loss.

Salt (Epsom and Regular)
Safety Issues: People with limited sodium intake should see a doctor before using any treatments using salt. May cause water retention.

Especially useful for soaks. Infections, sore muscles, sore throats, painful gums, sinus infections, allergies, poison ivy.

Tincture Bases

Keep a supply of Vodka on hand to make herbal tinctures. We use about 3 bottles per year.

If you are making Snakejuice*, then you will also need one bottle of Blackberry Brandy, and one bottle of Peppermint Schnapps per year.

Chapter Two

Essential Oils

Do not take essential oils by mouth. They are highly concentrated substances and in large amounts they can do internal damage.

If you are pregnant, any oils you use on yourself for massage or in the bath should be very weak dilutions. If you make any of the blends in this book, you should use half the stated number of drops. You are advised to use only the flower and fruit oils as they are very gentle. It is a good idea to consult a qualified homeopathic doctor or an aromatherapist for advice.

Skin Safety: Before applying oils to the skin, they should always be diluted in a carrier oils, such as sweet almond, olive, or coconut, because they are so concentrated. Anyone who doesn't have sensitive skin; ie. allergic reactions, Lavender or Tea tree may be used undiluted for first aid purposes (2 drops applied to the affected area.) If you are sensitive to nuts, use Olive oil instead.

If you massage an oil with a citrus blend into your skin, be aware that they contain a substance that can cause a skin reaction to UV light or sunlight. Be sure to avoid strong UV lights up to 12 hours after application.

Babies, Children, and Elderly: Correct dosages are critical because of the delicate skin of small children and the elderly.

Babies up to 2 years: One drop in 4 teaspoons of carrier oil for general skin and massage.

Children 2-10: Any blends made should contain half the stated number of drops.

Over the age of 10 may use the same dilutions as adults.

Elderly skin: In cases where the skin is delicate and thin where veins are visible, you should half the stated number of drops.

There are approximately 20 drops of Essential oil per ml.

Frankincense
Safety issues: None

Uses: Disinfects and heals cuts, wounds, eczema, and damaged skin; tones and rejuvenates mature skin, eases chesty coughs or bronchitis, comforts anxiety or emotional stress.

Garlic
Safety Issues: Do not use with blood thinners, birth control pills, some medications,

Used for high blood pressure, low blood pressure, infections, high cholesterol, coronary disease, prostate cancer, colon cancer, bladder cancer, osteoarthritis, flu and Swine flu, tick repellent, and yeast infections. Garlic is also used for earaches, menstrual disorders, stomach ulcers caused by H. pylori infection, exercise performance, fibrocystic breast disease.

Other uses include treatment of fever, coughs, headache, stomach ache, sinus congestion, gout, joint pain, hemorrhoids, asthma, bronchitis, shortness of breath, snakebites, diarrhea and bloody diarrhea, bloody urine, diphtheria, and whooping cough.

Some people apply garlic oil to their skin or nails to treat fungal infections, warts, and corns. It is also applied to the skin for hair loss and thrush.

Lavender
Safety issues: None

Uses: Soothes cuts, burns, wounds, insect bites, sore skin, eases headaches, tension, migraines, insomnia, anxiety. Useful for children and adults.

Myrrh
Safety issues: Myrrh is best avoided during pregnancy

Uses: Heals and disinfects deep cuts, wounds, chapped and cracked skin, eczema, cleans and disinfects the mouth easing sore gums and mouth ulcers, relieves bronchitis, chesty coughs, calms highly anxious emotional states.

Peppermint
Safety Issues: Be careful using peppermint with certain drugs as it may increase side effects of the medication.

Used for Irritable bowel syndrome, Indigestion, heartburn, respiratory issues, painkiller. Inflammation of the mouth and throat, colds, coughs, morning sickness. Mosquito repellent.

Tea Tree (Melaleuca)
Safety issues: Safe to use neat on the skin except on individuals with sensitive or allergy prone skin for whom it must be diluted in a carrier oil.

Uses: Clears skin infections and acne, heals wounds and cuts, soothes insect bites, clears athletes foot, helps with influenza, colds, bronchitis, and boosts general immunity.

Chapter Three
DEFINITIONS

Compress- A compress is a piece of cloth soaked in a bowl of hot or cold herbal treatments. Almost any herb can be applied as a compress. Cheesecloth or a pad made of lint or flannel are excellent choices for a compress.

Infusion- Warm a teapot and add about ¼ cup of dried herbs or ½ cup of fresh herbs. Pour 2/14 cups of hot water on the herbs. Cover the pot until the herbs have infused (about 10 minutes). Strain the infusion. Add a little honey if desired. May be kept in fridge up to 48 hours.

Massage Balm- Remedies in Olive oil base, ready for massage.

Steam Inhalation- Best for stressed or inflamed lungs, make up an infusion of the herb you want to use and add it to a basinful of hot water. A couple of drops of essential oils may be used as well. Drape a towel around your head and the basin so that you keep the steam in and inhale slowly and deeply for a few minutes.

Oils- . Take a quart jar and stuff it full of the herb you desire to make an oil of. Pour Olive oil over the entire batch, leaving enough airspace to shake it comfortably. Cap tightly. Leave in the sun, shaking 3x day for 3 days. Strain, and repeat using the same oil until you have reached the strength desired. Store in refrigerator. These are not as strong as distilled oils, but still work wonderfully well.

Tincture- An alcohol based medicine.

To make a tincture to drink hot or cold find a glass jar. Add about 1 3/4 cup of dried herbs or 4-5 cups of fresh herbs. Pour 2 ¼ cups of vodka (preservative). Add a scant cup of water seal the jar and store in a cool place for 2-3 weeks, checking and shaking it occasionally. Strain the liquid through a cheese cloth into sterilized bottles. Will keep up to a year.

Tea: Place 1 Tablespoon of dried leaves, in a cup of hot water and let steep. If using fresh herbs, use 2-3 sprigs. The longer it sits the stronger it is, but it may also become bitter.

Ointment: A mixture of an oil base, such as Olive, beeswax, and essential oils or herbs.

Chapter Four

General list of Antibiotics

Resistance to antibiotics is becoming a worldwide problem. That is the reason we use herbals medications as well as infection controls, such as handwashing and tooth brushing where possible. Diseases have very little resistance to herbal remedies.

General principals of antibiotic use:

- Only use antibiotics for general bacterial infections if there is a high risk of complications, symptoms aren't resolving, or symptoms are severe or significant.

- Use first line antibiotics (first choice) before attempting broad spectrum.

One of the most important things you can do if you are choosing to learn about which antibiotics work for which issues, is to pick up a Physican's Desk Reference. These contain information on diseases, doses for adults and children, as well as side effects, and things that would interfere with the actions of each drug. Another good reference book is the Nurses Drug Book. Get the most current title.

Respiratory infections to include Upper Respiratory (sinus and throat), COPD, Ear infections, Sinusitis. Urinary Tract infections

FIRST CHOICE: Amoxicillin
SECOND CHOICE: Ciprofloxacin

Lower Respiratory (Bronchitis, Pneumonia), soft tissue (wounds and abcesses), Bones,
FIRST CHOICE: Cephalexin (Keflex)

Whooping Cough, Chlamydia, Gonorrhea, Urethritis

FIRST CHOICE: Azythromycin

Oral infections, acne
FIRST CHOICE: Clindamyacin

Ear infections, bladder infections, and E. Coli or salmonella infection.
FIRST CHOICE: Amoxicillin or Ampicillin WARNING: DO NOT USE if you are allergic to Penicillin.

SECOND CHOICE: Ciprofloxacin

Severe infections of the Urinary tract, lower repiratory, skin, bone, joint, stomach, sinuses, and prostate.
FIRST CHOICE: Ciprofloxacin

Infections that cause Stomach ulcers, Lyme disease, Anthrax (in conjuction with other medications)
FIRST CHOICE: Tetracycline

Dosages for Adults

Amoxicillin: 500mg every 12 hours. For SEVERE infections: 500mg every 8 hrs
Ampicillin: 500mg every 12 hours
Azithromycin (Z-pack): 500mg the first day, 250mg per day for 4 more days.
Cephalexin (Keflex): 500mg every 12 hours

Ciprofloxacin: 500, 750, or 1000mg once a day
Clindamycin: 450mg every 6 hours
Tetracycline: 500mg every 6 hours for 14-30 days

Chapter Five

RECIPES

ALLERGIES

Local Raw honey in your area is one of the best remedies for allergies. To develop immunities to the pollens in your area drink Chamomile tea, which is a natural antihistamine, mixed with local honey to help with allergies.

Raw garlic chopped and eaten helps with asthma and hay fever. We chop raw garlic, and mix with 2 TB of olive oil, sea salt, and a little black pepper. Dip French bread and eat daily to help keep up immunities and help with asthma.

Simmer chopped fresh cabbage leaves in hot water for about 5 minutes, strain and drink the liquid.

Take a cup of apple cider vinegar, bring to a boil with two chopped cloves of garlic and simmer for a few minutes. Strain and add one TB of raw honey. Drink.

Eucalyptus oil in hot water to make a steam is a good inhalation treatment for asthma. Place 5 drops of Eucalyptus oil in a basin of hot water. Place a clean dish towel over your head to make a steam tent. Breathe in steam.

To ease breathing, prop up patient in a 45 degree angle to help open lung passages. Take 3 drops of Eucalyptus oil and 3 drops of Peppermint oil. Rub small amount underneath nose or on patients chest to ease breathing.

BURNS

Mild first degree burns are usually able to be treated at home, If a patient has second or third degree burns, they should be transported to medical attention as soon as possible.

The first thing to do with burn at home is to cool it down by running it under cool running water. If the burn is chemical in nature, keep flushing the skin with cold running water, for 10 minutes until it stops hurting.

For first degree burns, we use lavender oil that we make ourselves with olive oil. (see recipe)

Apple cider vinegar soothes burns as well. This works especially well on sunburns.

Aloe Vera has been long known for its uses in burn treatment. We take Aloe Vera, a little raw honey, some plain yogurt and mash it all together. This works well.

BLEEDING

Yarrow Tincture to stop bleeding:
1 tsp of Yarrow tincture to 1/2 cup water Put on cloth and press on wound.

In a pinch, white flour or cornstarch will help a wound coagulate quickly.

FEVERS

A fever is not necessarily a bad thing. It's the bodies way of destroying harmful bacteria and infections. Fevers that go on for long periods of time are another story.

To cool a person with a high fever, place cool wet cloths in the patients armpits, groin area and back of the neck to bring down the fever. Wiping down areas of the body with cool cloths will also encourage evaporation on the skin which will help cool the patient down as well.

A patient may also be placed in a bath with lukewarm or barely cool water. It is important to use lukewarm or tepid water, not cold, as the temperature difference could cause the patient to go into shock. As the temperature comes down, you may use cooler water.

Apple cider vinegar and honey made into a tea, will work at lowering a fever.

URINARY TRACT INFECTIONS

1. Lemons and cream of tartar

    1½ tsp of cream of tartar

    Fresh lemon juice

    Water

2. Ginger tea

3. 2 Tb apple cider vinegar in glass of water. Drink 2x day.

    3. Chop 2-3 raw onions and boil in as many cups of water. Drink the water over the course of the day to help with Urinary tract infections.

EYE INFECTION

1. Chamomile tea

    1 cup Hot water

    1 tsp Raw Honey

Steep 2 tea bags in hot water for 15 minutes. Let tea cool. This is important before adding raw honey, as heat kills the medicinal benefits. Add raw honey and stir until dissolved. Place drops of cooled mixture to affected eye 2x-3x day for 3 days, or until symptoms completely resolved. Store remainder in the refrigerator in a covered container for up to 3 days.

2. Raw Apple Cider Vinegar (with the Mother)

    1 Tablespoon of ACV to one cup of water. Dab onto eyes with a cotton ball.

3. Lactating mothers may use breast milk in the eye.

NASAL DECONGESTION

1 cup tomato juice
½ tsp hot sauce or pinch of cayenne pepper
1 tsp lemon juice
pinch of salt or celery salt
1 tsp fresh garlic.

2. Chew 3-4 Black Peppercorns.

SINUS OR RESPIRATORY INFECTION

Ginger Root and Pineapple Juice.
Take one or two arms off a Ginger root. Chop and put in 2 cups of water. Bring to a simmer. Do not boil. Turn off heat and let sit for 15 minutes. Let cool. Pour water into a cup. Match 1:1 with pineapple juice. Drink one cup in morning, and one cup at night. Do not exceed three days of treatment without a break in between.

EAR INFECTION

2 cloves of fresh garlic chopped
5 TB olive oil

Soak garlic in olive oil for 15 minutes. Warm (SLIGHTLY) and making sure drops are not hot, place a few drops of strained oil into affected ear. Put in a cotton ball to prevent drips. Repeat up to 3x day for 3 days or until infection is gone. Store in refrigerator.

TOPICAL STAPH INFECTIONS OR BLEPHERITIS

Make an oil with ¼ tsp ground cloves and ¼ tsp of ground cinnamon in 3 Tbs of Olive oil. Let set in oil 15 minutes or overnight (better). Alternate the cinnamon/clove oil with Lavender oil every other time.

Colloidal silver will help with MRSA or Staph.

Essential Oils that help with MRSA and Staph:
Oil of Oregano, Thyme, Cinnamon, and Tea Tree.

MRSA and Staph Infections- apply with Q-tip or spray with spray bottle over wound.

BLEPHERITIS- Wash affected lid with baby soap, dry and then apply lavender oil first. Wait 5 minutes and then apply the Clove/Cinnamon oil with a Q tip. Do not get in the eye itself as it will sting. Repeat 2-3 times a day until resolved. At first sign of recurrence, apply again. Oil may be kept in refrigerator up to three days for reuse.

SHOCK

Sugar has been used to offset the symptoms of shock for years. If a person is experiencing mild shock or anxiety, give one cup of hot chamomile tea with honey. Orange Juice also works well.

TOOTHACHE

Apply ¼ tsp cloves to 2 Tbs Olive oil to sore teeth, or infected gums. Swish and spit.

NOSEBLEEDS
If you get a nosebleed that won't stop, drink a cup of Peppermint tea..this will help clot blood immediately.

Oregano oil, Clove oil, Tea Tree Oil, Cinnamon oil, Thyme oil

JVJ (VOODOO JUICE)
For Flu and Cold, Sinus and Respiratory

Boil 1 quart of water
Add 4 arms of fresh chopped ginger

Simmer for 15 minutes, then turn off heat. Let sit 10 minutes. Pour water into a container, mix 50:50 with pineapple juice. Drink 1 cup in am, and 1 cup pm for three days.

BRONCHITIS AND ASTHMA

1 quart of water
1 Tbs dried basil leaves
1 tsp ginger powdered
Honey and Lemon to taste

Boil water, pull off heat add ginger and basil leaves. Let steep 15 minutes. Add honey and fresh lemon juice just before drinking

ELDERBERRY COLD AND FLU SYRUP

Take a quart jar and fill with *dried* elderberries. Pour Vodka over the berries, until covered. Cover jar, and store in a cool dry place for 2 months, shaking daily. Strain and store.

ELDERBERRY COUGH SYRUP

Homemade Elderberry Syrup Ingredients:

2/3 cup black elderberries
3.5 cups of water
2 T fresh or dried ginger root
1 tsp cinnamon powder
1/2 tsp cloves or clove powder
1 cup raw honey (we get from our farmer's market)
How to Make Elderberry Syrup:

Pour water into medium saucepan and add elderberries, ginger, cinnamon and cloves (do not add honey!)

Bring to a boil and then cover and reduce to a simmer for about 45 minutes to an hour until the liquid has reduced by almost half. At that point, remove from heat and let cool enough to be handled. Pour through a strainer into a glass jar or bowl.

Discard the elderberries (or compost them!) and let the liquid cool to lukewarm. When it is no longer hot, add 1 cup of honey and stir well.

When honey is well mixed into the elderberry mixture, pour the syrup into a pint sized mason jar or 16 ounce glass bottle of some kind.

Standard dose : ½-1 tsp for kids and ½ - 1 Tbsp for adults. Take the normal dose every 2-3 hours instead of once a day if cold is in process.

MIGRAINE TINCTURE

3 parts lemon balm
2 parts feverfew
vodka

Put desired amounts of chopped herbs in a quart jar, and cover with vodka. Cap, and put in a sunny place, shaking 2x day for 4-6 weeks. Strain and pour tincture into clean glass jar. Store up to 3 years in a dark colored bottle. Dosage for adults is ¼ to ½ teaspoon of the tincture every thirty minutes to one hour until symptom subsides.

COLD SORES/HERPES SORES

Drink 1 cup of Licorice tea in the morning and one in the evening. Place the used cooled tea bag over cold sore for 5-10 minutes each time.

Lemon Balm, Echinacea, Black Coffee, or Raw Honey.

SNAKE JUICE

Uses: Colds, Flu, H1N1, Plague, Respiratory

Take a gallon jar, layer sliced yellow onions, and lemons until full. Pour raw honey over until covered. Add one bottle Blackberry brandy, and one bottle Peppermint schnapps. Let sit in cool dark place for 3 months, shaking occasionally. Strain and store in dark colored bottle up to one year. Use for colds, Flu, H1N1

JOCK ITCH

Oil of Oregano, diluted with olive oil. If it doesn't go away within a day or so, use undiluted.

HEART ATTACKS

Useful in stopping heart attacks if there are no other options available. Some physicians swear it is as effective as Nitroglycerin at stopping heart issues.

Cayenne Pepper Tea.

Take one cup of hot water and add 1 tsp of cayenne pepper, or take a few droppers of Cayenne tincture. African Bird Pepper is the best. This has been known to stop heart attacks in under 3 minutes. Every first aid kit should have a small bottle of Cayenne Tincture.

SHOULD NOT BE TAKEN WITH ACE INHIBITORS

Cayenne Tincture Recipe
1 cup Cayenne pepper to 2 cups Vodka
Place in jar and store in cool dark place.
Shake well 2x day for 3-4 weeks. Strain. Keep in cool dark place.

Dosage for adults: Place 5-15 drops in a cup of hot water or tea. Take up to 3x day. This tincture is extremely hot. The older the Cayenne peppers (if you use real ones) the hotter the tincture.

HOT TIGER BALM

Melt Beeswax and coconut oil 1 oz beeswax to ¼ cup coconut or olive oil.
10 drops camphor essential oil
 9 drops peppermint essential oil
 7 drops eucalyptus essential oil
 5 drops clove essential oil
 5 drops cinnamon essential oil to the melted beeswax mixture, and quickly stir.

Complete this step before the beeswax cools and hardens, because it will be difficult to add the essential oils at that point

HERBAL MESS

My family scoffs at my homeopathic treatments. I get a lot of eye rolling and "uh huhs" from people other than my children, because they know they work....here is our dog's treatment from

the last two weeks. She had been missing for a couple of days, and when we found her, the wound was unable to be stitched, it was too old. I did treat it myself, as the vet wanted almost $800. The wound was over 6 inches long. I could put my whole hand it. It took two weeks and this was the result...Using ONLY my homeopathic herbal mess, 10 menstrual pads, a pair of nylons, some sheets, and a girdle we picked up from Good will...Entire cost of treatment, under $5.00. She was kept in a kennel and taken outside under supervision so she didn't tear them ...tape didn't work, superglue worked for a short time, but she kept tearing the nylons off and reopening it.

Recipe

Mix equal parts raw honey and olive oil. Add ¼ cup chopped Comfrey. Add layers, don't remove previous layers. Cover with gauze and wrap.

The first pic is 2-3 days old, before treatment.

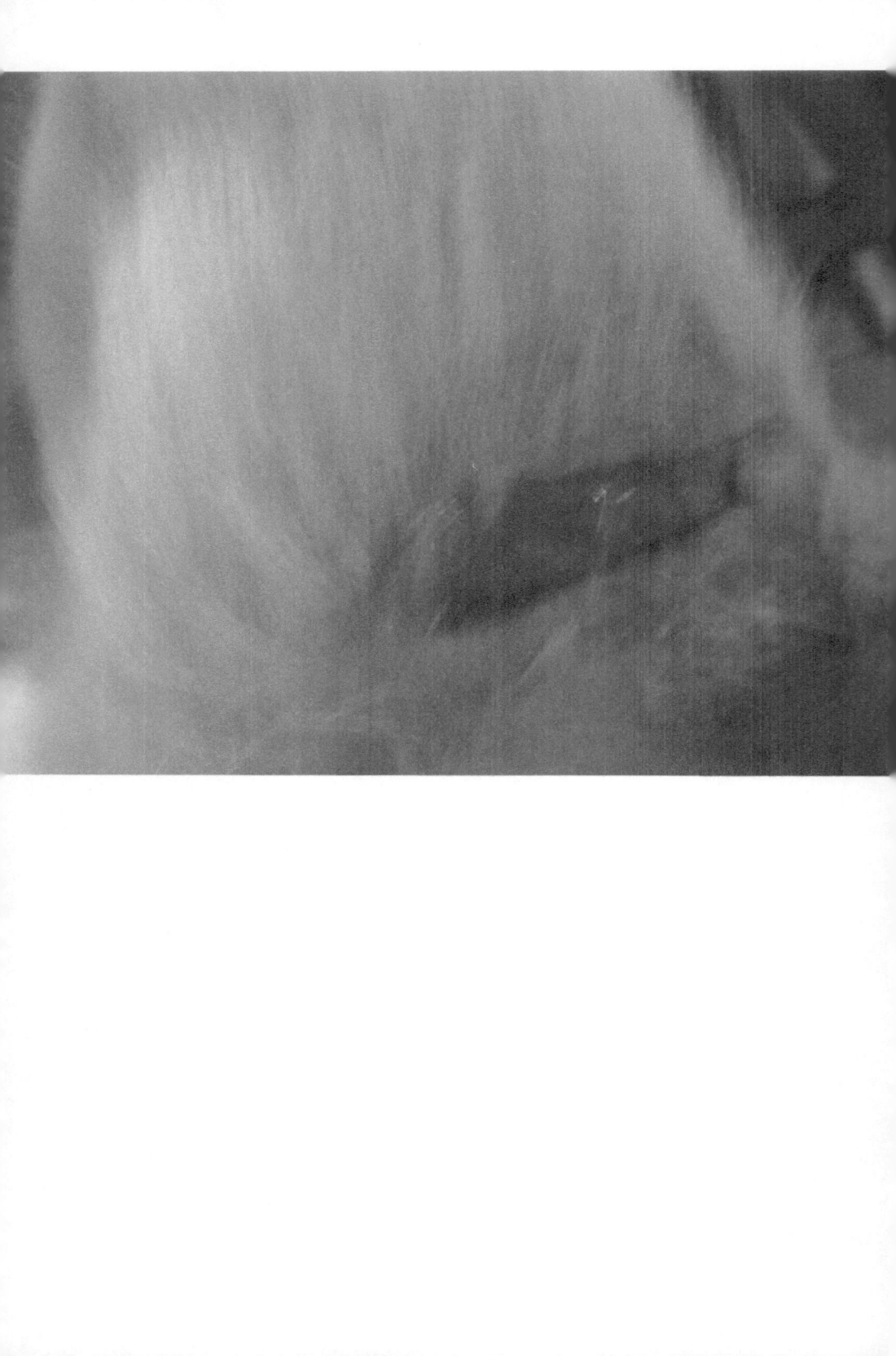

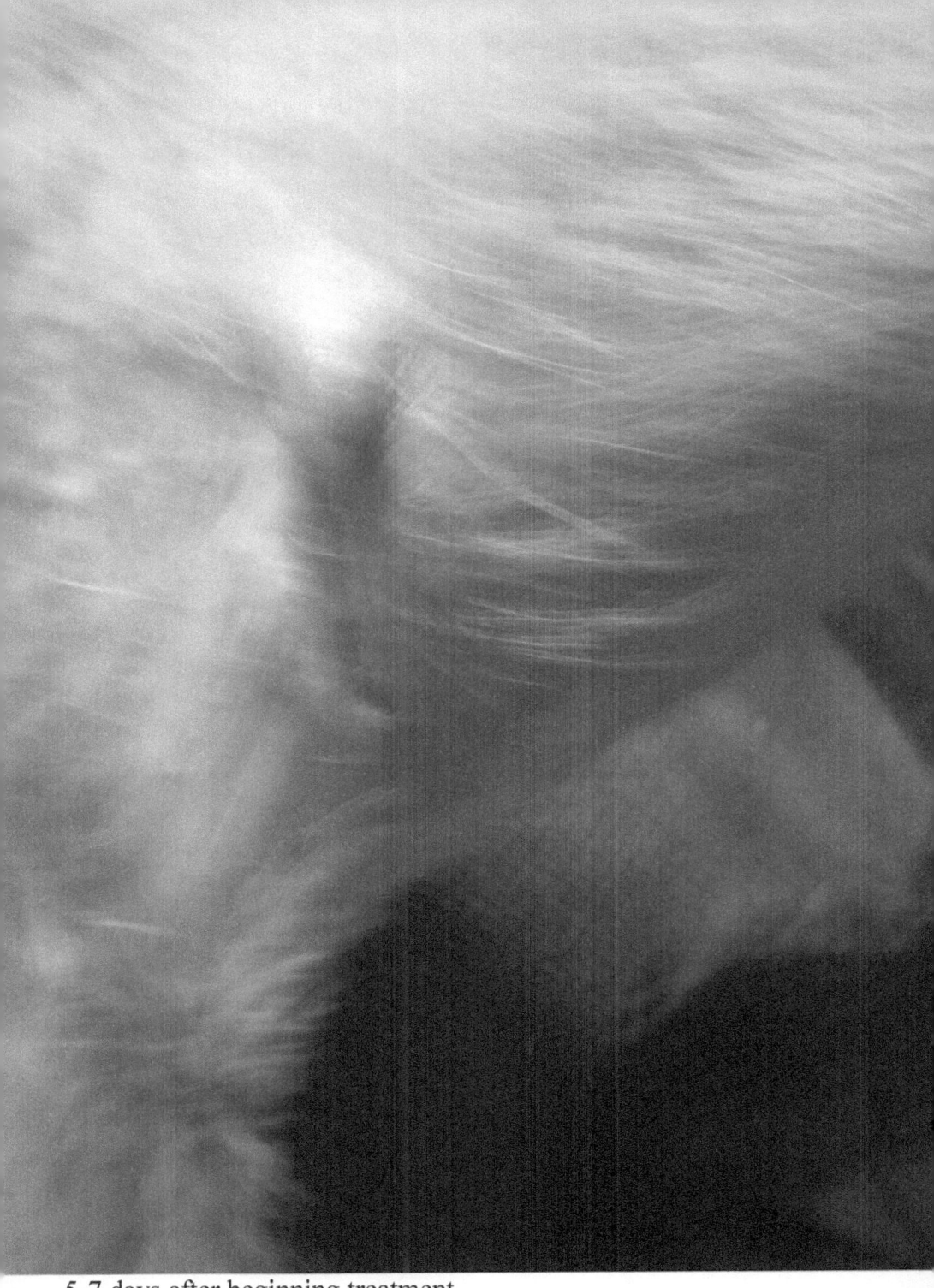
5-7 days after beginning treatment.

The last one was about day 10. Yesterday I looked at it and there is no scar, no lump nothing to tell it had been there except no hair.

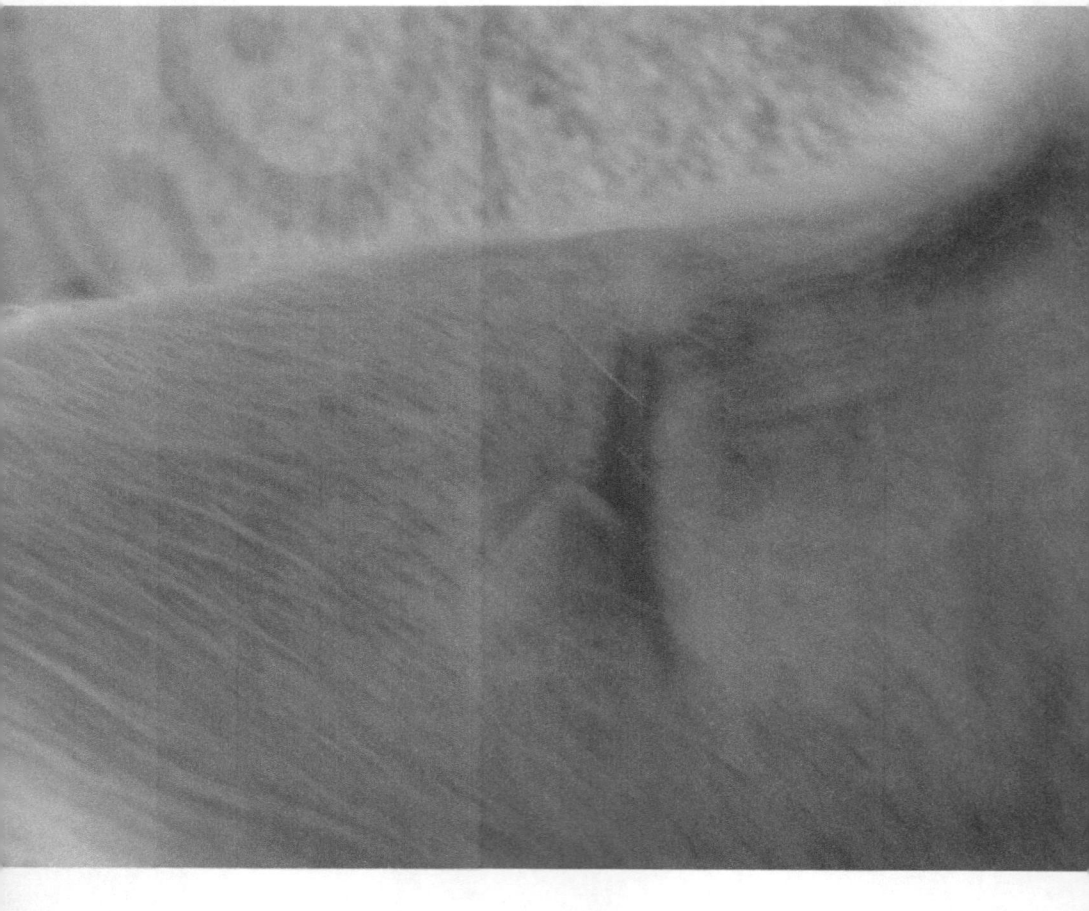

CHARCOAL POULTICE

To make a charcoal poultice, you will need the following items:

Activated charcoal powder
Water
Some type of soft cloth such as gauze

Mix two to three tablespoons of activated charcoal powder with a small amount of water. Add just enough water to make a spreadable paste.
Spread the paste over a layer of gauze, lint or flannel.
Cover the paste with another layer of material so that the charcoal and water mixture is between the two pieces of material.
Place the poultice over the injured body part, taking care to make sure that material covers the entire area.
Place plastic wrap over the top of the poultice, and wrap with an Ace bandage or cloth strip and then secure.
Leave in place for up to ten hours, replacing as necessary when it dries.
Adding a few tablespoons of oatmeal to the charcoal/water paste can help retain moisture.

SAFETY ISSUES

Serious injuries, illness, inflammations and sprains need medical attention. Before you self-treat serious illness or injury, visit your personal health care provider for appropriate treatment.

If you are treating an area with mucous membranes, such as your eye, use a less porous cloth than gauze, such as a towel.

Never reuse the poultices...always make a fresh one.

Do not apply charcoal poultices to open wounds. If charcoal gets into an open wound, it will leave a permanent mark on your skin.

DRY MUSTARD PLASTER

Besides being used as a painkiller for backache, mustard plasters were also used to treat coughs and infections of the chest and lungs. A mustard plaster works by creating heat, drawing toxins out of the body through the skin.

1 part dry mustard powder
3 Parts Whole Wheat Flour

Add enough water to make it into a paste a little thinner than pancake batter.
Place between a piece of flannel material, or towels. Spread paste on one half and fold the other half over.

DO NOT LET IT COME IN CONTACT WITH SKIN.

The ratio of mustard powder to flour will determine how much heat the plaster will give, and therefore how often it will need to be checked to make sure it is not burning the skin and whether or not it can be used overnight, on a child or on sensitive skin.

1:8 Very weak, safe overnight (1/4 teaspoon mustard powder to 2 teaspoons flour)
1:6 Mild, suitable for children, safe overnight for adult with normal skin. (Mix 1/2 teaspoon of mustard seed powder with 1 tablespoon of flour. Should cover a 6"x6" square area.)
1:4 Strong. Good for relieving chest congestion due to colds, use only during day or set alarm clock if using at night.
1:3 Very strong. Adults only, not suitable for children. Check frequently for signs of redness.

Making sure the skin is dry, place the plaster on the desired area. Check frequently to make sure there is no allergic reaction. Remove when skin begins to turn red, usually after 10-20 minutes using a 1:4 ratio. Do not leave on any longer than 30 minutes at a time. After removing the plaster it is best if the person can remain in bed and sleep for a couple hours. May be repeated after 2 hours, up to 3 times a day.

Do not place directly against skin. It will burn.

If it burns on application, remove immediately. Change every 4-6 hours as needed.

TURBERCULOSIS (TB)

TB is a bacterial infection of the lungs. The symptoms get worse with time. At first, there will be a hacking, barking cough, which turns into chest pains and coughing up blood. Other symptoms are chills, fever, night sweats, loss of appetite and weight loss. TB can sit in your system for years and popping up when you least expect it. It is contagious and airborne. It is spread by coughing, sneezing, spitting, kissing, and contact with discharged mucus.

Once again, I am NOT a doctor, and I don't claim to be. The following information is a place to start, if you are interested in looking into alternative treatments for these diseases. That being said, we use Naturopathic remedies at our home with fantastic results most of the time. Every treatment will react differently to every body, because of the personal makeup of that person's genetic background. Find what works for you and stick with it.

Tuberculosis is curable and one needs to remember that at all times. With proper care and management, the disease can be completely cured and the person can go back to leading a normal life.

TREATMENTS FOR TB

A glass of freshly-squeezed orange juice with a pinch of salt, a spoonful of honey, and two-three mint leaves, should be mixed and given to the patient. The saline effect in the lungs will reduce expectoration and protect the patient from other secondary infections.

Vitamin C contained in orange juice boosts the immune system.

Regular intake of Pineapple juice breaks up congestion in the chest. One of our recipes calls for Ginger root boiled and the water mixed with Pineapple juice for chest congestion. This really works.

Crystallized sugar dipped in Clove oil, taken in small amounts helps the symptoms..

Garlic

Garlic has been found to be effective in treating tuberculosis. In fact, garlic is an amazing antimicrobial herb which works effectively against microbes, harmful organisms, bacteria, fungi, parasites and viruses.

This makes garlic a critical part of any tuberculosis home remedy or natural treatment.

An ideal way to go about preparing the medication would be to boil 30 garlic cloves in 150 ml of milk mixed in 50 ml of water. This entire portion should be boiled until it condenses to 50 ml of concentrated garlic syrup. After filtering, the concentrated syrup free from solid substances should be administered to the patient twice daily.

Do note that a good quality garlic bulb should have 10 to 12 large, white cloves. Garlic bulbs with many small or yellowish cloves are probably of inferior quality. For best effect, use garlic that is organic and raw.

Herbal Tea

Licorice root tea prepared with only licorice or with other herbs like sage and chamomile in equal quantities can prove very effective for throat pain and providing relief from persistent coughing. All these herbs are effective in treating respiratory conditions.

Mint is another useful supplement in a treatment for tuberculosis.

A glass of fresh mint tea mixed with 1 cup of carrot juice, two spoons of honey and malt vinegar.

The juice can be administered 3x daily since it dissolves the mucus, cleans the lungs, develops immunity, acts as a detoxifying agent and cleanses the body of all anti-tuberculosis drug side effects.

American ginseng

After consulting a pediatrician or physician, children with tuberculosis can be administered American ginseng three times a day.

Ginseng contains minerals and nutrients that help build immunity and increase the bodies resistance to other infections and diseases.

In addition to all of the above, persons suffering from TB need to get a lot of exposure to sunshine, nutritious food, exercise, and should drink plenty of water to help in the detoxification process.

HOMEMADE ELECTROLYTE SOLUTION

6-8 tsp raw molasses to ½ tsp salt in one quart of water. Drink ¼-1/2 cup 2x day for rehydration, or diarrhea. Do not mix in fruit juice.

Measure ingredients carefully as too much sugar or too much salt, can worsen the diarrhea.

IMMUNE BOOST

Garlic is effective against at least 30 types of bacteria, viruses, parasites and fungi. It has anti-inflammatory and astringent properties.

Echinacea and Goldenseal boosts your immune system.

Immune System Booster Tea
2 cups of water.
1 tsp. Echinacea root.
½ tsp. Chamomile leaves.
½ tsp. Peppermint leaves.
Combine all these ingredients. If you have evidence of a depressed immune system, take 3 tsp. of the formula daily for up to 5 days. Double the dose during an infection.

WOUNDS AND INFECTIONS

Test oils on the inside skin of arm to see if there is an allergic reaction before using. Most people don't have reactions to essential oils, but check to make sure. People who have sensitive skin dilute with oils and water before use.

Wash any cuts with witch hazel to prevent infection. If none is available saltwater or water with lemon juice will work...it stings but works well.

In your choice of carrier oil, mix:

10 drops tea tree oil

10 drops Lavender oil

5 drops each of Myrhh, Frankincense, and Chamomile oil.

Shake well. Add to 1 cup of water in a spray bottle and shake well. Spray on open wound 2x daily until resolved. Wound may appear red afterwards up to 10 minutes after spraying, this is normal. If redness continues longer, discontinue.

THIEVES OIL

Bubonic plague outbreaks decimated the population of Asia and Europe for the better part of a thousand years. A legend appeared of four thieves that were captured and charged with robbing the dead and dying victims. When the thieves were in court the magistrate offered leniency if they would reveal how they resisted the infection as they robbed the plague dead. They told of a special concoction of aromatic herbs, including garlic, cloves and rosemary, that they rubbed on themselves before committing their crimes. Found to reduce airborne bacteria by 99.96%

Topical or Inhalation

Supports the immune system and respiratory infections

40 drops Clove Bud essential oil
35 drops Lemon essential oil
20 drops Cinnamon Bark essential oil
15 drops Eucalyptus essential oil
10 drops Rosemary essential oil –

Conclusion

I firmly believe that as Preppers we have a responsibility to ourselves, our family, and to others who may need help. I hope this book gives you ideas to pursue, to increase your herbal knowledge, if all else fails. I have seen fantastic results, but it is for you to decide whether it works for you or not.

Be safe.

www.ingramcontent.com/pod-product-compliance
Lightning Source LLC
Chambersburg PA
CBHW031557210526
45464CB00003B/1320